BAREFOOT AGAIN

Living Without Neuropathy!

By

Roxanne DeLillo

Dedicated to All of you, who are fighting to eradicate neuropathy from your life. May your journey bring you relief from numbness, pain, burning and tingling. I hope you find joy in walking Barefoot Again!

A Special "Thank You," to Ben, for his help and input, with the writing of this book. Your positive outlook on life, and your way of seeing the humor in the face of dealing with this disease, was truly inspiring for me. Thanks again, from the bottom of my heart!

Forward – v

Chapter One - Nothing You Can Do! 1

Chapter Two - Something I Can Do 10

Chapter Three - They're Amputating My Foot! 27

Chapter Four - The Pain is Unbearable 31

Chapter Five - Haven't Felt My Feet in 20 Years 40

Chapter Six - What It's All About 45

Chapter Seven - What Does it all Mean? 50

Chapter Eight - Myths and My Opinion 64

Chapter Nine - Where do you start? 70

Chapter Ten - The Light Bulb Comes On! 72

Chapter Eleven - At Home, On Your Own 84

Chapter Twelve - Get the Gunk Out 96

Chapter Thirteen - Changing for the Better 105

Chapter Fourteen - You Can Do This! 116

Resources, Routines & Restrictions 118

Contraindications 133

Foot Map 142

Forward

Her smile swept over me like a warm summer breeze. I was so shocked that I didn't quite know how to respond! My wife saved the day and introduced us. "Hi, I'm Emily and this is my husband, Ben." Emily sent me a sidewise glance, with a little smirk on her face. I lost that bet! I guess I better explain. You see, for years I had not felt my feet, well, that is except for the incessant burning pain, and, the constant feel of ants eating my feet from the inside out! Yes, my feet were like walking on wooden pegs, that had a mind of their own. Ever try balancing on wooden pegs? Not easy! Sometimes I thought my brain was numb too.

And did I mention the stumbling and imbalance? The sluggish body and loopy head from my drug pusher, I mean, doctor, had become the norm for me. Yes, I was a wreck! I had been to countless, and I mean, countless, doctors and therapists, over the years. Some promised to help, but, it would take time and cost me a pretty penny, as insurance wouldn't pay. The only promise they kept was taking my money, I guess they didn't lie about that part.

So, this search for some relief and not seeing any results, left me quite pessimistic to any more "help." I was what you would call "jaded." I wasn't going to go easy on the next money grabber I was told to go see, by another good intentioned friend. I made a bet with my wife, that the next office we went to, would be like all the others. Front desk receptionist would put on a fake smile, look up, just long enough to tell me to fill out the one-hundred-page questionnaire and bring it back up when done. Then I would sit for five hours, waiting to see a doctor or therapist for about 15 minutes, (they are generous with their time on the first visit), then either be prescribed a million supplements or something else that wouldn't work, that I had already tried. Yes, you could say I was very "optimistic" about this visit today. I had grumbled during the drive over, but my wife, sweet thing that she is, helped me see the light, of trying one more time. She said she had heard this gal was different, and that she never kept you waiting. I bet her a steak dinner at the restaurant of her choice, if this gal greeted us. I'd even wear my best suit, if this gal gave us a smile that didn't say, "I want your money." I knew I had her at that one. Even she couldn't argue that we had spent a fortune over the last several years, with no results. That is the reason behind my wife's smirk!

I will say, it took me by complete surprise to have Roxanne, herself, not a receptionist, greet us with a smile and look us straight in the eye, like she was actually glad to see us! She asked if we would like to use the restroom or wanted some water, as this was going to take a while. She said she had a ten-page intake form, that we would be filling out together, over the next hour or two. "Sometimes this can take a little longer, depending upon how much you have abused your body, so it may take two and a half hours. Don't worry, I always block out time for it to run over, but the price is the same." What? I didn't have to fill it out? She was going to do the paperwork, not her assistant? I lost that bet too! Had to bring my wife breakfast in bed for a week over that one. Not sure I like this gal! She is costing me way too much already.

The time seemed to fly by during the intake. She asked many questions, that nobody had ever asked. We also got to drill her, I was a Drill Sergeant at one time, about what she was going to do for me. I will have to tell you, this was the first time I ever left an office, with hope in my heart! She even hugged us both goodbye and said she looked forward to seeing me next week! "Don't worry, this will get better," she said. My wife adopted her, right then and there!

She said I would need to come in Monday through Friday, for two weeks. Emily and I discussed how different this time was, over dinner at Ruth Chris. Yes, she picked one of the pricey places!

Now I'm not going to take you through all the treatments, however, I will tell you that by the end of the first week, all my pain was gone! By the end of the second, I had feeling in both feet and I was walking barefoot around my house! Now I am just trying to find the right cruise to the Bahamas. Yes, you guessed it, I lost another bet! My wife mentioned something about putting her in our will!

I worked with Roxanne a little, well, gave my input, regarding the home treatments she talks about in here. She would explain to me what a person would need to do, to help themselves at home. I would then put myself in their place, and let her know if I thought it was doable. I think you will find that she has made it easy for you to do on your own. You will get improvement, if you follow what she tells you to do. It might sound like a lot, but, it really isn't. It is what needs to be done, to improve your symptoms of neuropathy. I know this does not take the place of being able to go through her treatment program, and takes a little longer, however, according to those that have tried this, (no, you aren't the first to do it alone,) it does get great results, sometimes even complete relief from all symptoms.

I hope you enjoy this book as much as I enjoyed being a part of it. This remarkable lady has given a priceless gift to all who suffer from neuropathy. Now, take a step towards your new life today, and read the rest of this wonderful book. Don't panic, I'm not leaving just yet, I have one more story to tell you, about how it all started for me, in the first chapter.

Happy Walking, Ben

Chapter One - Nothing You Can Do!

No, "Sorry!" I can't help, or empathy of any kind, just the flat statement, "Nothing you can do." The words sent chills down my spine. Just the thought of never getting rid of this horrible pain and numbness in my feet, froze me to the bone. Does my doctor even realize that he has just given me a mini heart attack with those words? My brain scrambles to interpret what he just said but I feel the numbness creeping into my skull and I can't think. "Ben? Ben? Are you listening to me?" I finally come back to reality and he proceeds to tell me that he is giving me a prescription to help with the pain. He says it may help with the burning, that never lets up. He tries to explain that the numbness will continue up my legs, which gives me a minor stroke, and that it is normal to feel the pain, even after they go numb. "You will have trouble with your balance and you will never be able to go barefoot again." He says nonchalantly. OK, now I know I am having a heart attack! You are telling me that I can never go barefoot on the beach or in my house, ever? My mind races back to all the days on the beach with my beautiful wife and all the tropical vacations we have planned. This is supposed to be our time together. This is when we get to spend all our children's inheritance. My mind snaps back just in time to hear him explaining to me that it will sort of feel like I am walking on sticks.

Of course, you will feel these sticks as far as the pain goes, but, you won't be able to feel where you are placing your foot. Yea, that makes perfect sense to me! I mumble a few short expletives to calm my nerves and he shoots me a look of disdain. Easy for him, he feels his feet! Bet he would say there is something he could do if HE got this. I ask God to transfer this neuropathy to him, you know, so it will help find a cure. Not that I am thinking of myself, this is for the benefit of all mankind!

These memories keep my mind busy while I sit, again, in my doctor's office, waiting to hear what he will tell me this time. I look around at everyone waiting with me and start adding in my head. He has five rooms, and he spends about 5 minutes with each of us. There are nine of us waiting for a chance to be blessed by his presence, and five are already in the rooms. I know it cost me $75 every time I come in, so he is doing pretty good, considering he hasn't actually helped many of us. It's a pretty sum of money, we have all paid, to probably hear the same thing. I think I could do as good a job as the doc does. Let's see, "You still don't feel your feet, it hurts, burns, yes, yes, same old story, here's a pill for you." Yup, I could do it. I finally got the privilege of seeing this all-knowing doctor, after he is late by about 40 minutes, I guess he thinks his time is worth more than mine. "Anything new this time?" he asks. "No, just seems a little more numb, then last time, and, the pain keeps me awake at night. My wife made me move to the guest bedroom so she could get some sleep." He shrugs his shoulders and says something along the line of that is to be expected because she needs her sleep too. He doesn't have a clue how much restraint it took for me, not to knock him off his high stool! I'm telling him that this is disrupting my marriage, and he passes it off as nothing. I happen to like sleeping with my wife. My mind goes for a trip outside of the room for a bit to clear my head. I finally come back into my body in time to hear him give me his time honed speech. "I know this isn't what you want to hear, however, since you haven't responded well to any of the previous drugs, I am going to put you on an antidepressant." What? I'm not depressed, well, except every time I talk with you! He says it helps when dealing with neuropathy. I'm starting to hate that word, him too. Then he hands me a piece of paper with a few neuropathy support groups on it. He says it would be good for me to finally listen to him, (I guess he mentioned this a few times before, must have been during one of my office strokes,) and find a group to share my troubles with. Now I don't know about you but the last thing I want to do is go listen to other people talking about their pain. I think the energy in the room with all of them would probably make me numb all over. I come back to my senses long enough to hear him say that he will see me in another six months. I ask him "Why"? He looks at me with the deer in the headlights look and says, "What do you mean, why?" I said, well, I have been coming to see you for over ten years now and you haven't done anything to truly help so far. You keep me on drugs that almost got me a divorce and one that almost lost me my job. Now you say there is nothing you can do to change the progression of this disease except more and more drugs to numb my brain. I was quite pleased with my rant and the look on his face now. Not so smug now, are you doctor! I told him I thought it was about time I started looking elsewhere as I finally realized, after a few "office strokes and heart attacks" that if I was going to get any real help, it was up to me. I let him know that I was done with him and that I was filing for a medical divorce! Yes, it felt like I had been in an abusive relationship for far too many years and that I needed to cut the strings. I think they call it something like codependence or something like that. I felt the rush of adrenalin as I told him he had taken enough of my time and money, with no positive results. I handed him back the paper with the group addresses and told him to go join one of these and listen to them. It might put a burr under his nether region to help find something that truly worked. He mumbled something under his breath, think it was close to what I was thinking earlier, and left the room. Awe, the power of taking my life back and stepping out into the world of exploration! I felt elated to finally be doing something, not just listening to the same old record! When I got home I called my wife and told her she could come home. I wasn't in a drug rage anymore.

Chapter Two - Something I Can Do

Let me go back and explain what got me to this point in my life, where I divorce my doctor. You see, I had been going to see my doctor for years. I thought that was the only choice I had. So, the codependence began. As I complained, he gave me drugs. First it was the tingling, he gave me a drug. Then it turned to burning, and he gave me another drug. Then I got deep cramping, and he gave me a stronger drug. Then I lost all the feeling in my feet and he tried another drug. Some of the drugs made me feel like my brain was numb, others made me tired, one made me nauseous and others have had various other side effects some that were about as bad as the neuropathy. With one of the drugs, name not mentioned here, don't need them chasing me down and sending me on a permanent vacation, I got one of the common side effects. Now that doesn't sound bad until you hear the side effect. It is double vision! Think of trying to decide which road to take, left or right, all the time. Not fun! Now I was also blessed with a few of the "Minor" side effects. I know, sounds like nothing, right? Well, let me tell you, it isn't nothing! Dizziness, vomiting and diarrhea! Not a great combination to say the least! So here I am, seeing double and must go to the bathroom. I'm thinking the burning in my feet isn't that bad after all. Maybe that is what they plan on when they prescribe it. Take your mind off your real problem. Another one of the drugs gave me the gift of more than one side effect. This one almost cost me my job. My first side effect gift was clumsiness or unsteadiness. Now this may not sound that bad, however when you stumble around the office, they tend to think you have been taking an extra-long lunch. Then, when the other side effect kicks in; slurred speech along with the emotional side effects of; reacting too quickly, too emotional, or overreacting, comes into play, you just look guilty. Let's just say, it took a lot of convincing and a letter from my doctor, not to lose my job.

Now my wife is a saint, really, she is. She has been by my side with encouraging words, for years.

After changing the previous drug to another one, doc said it would save the day, I found out just how far a saint's patience will go. You see, not only did it give me the gift of a few fun side effects, it gave me one that any wife will tell you is beyond annoying! Uncontrolled back-and-forth and/or rolling eye movements. Yes, you heard me, rolling eye movements. I didn't realize this was starting to be part of my body function until my wife asked me if her new outfit looked good. Well, I guess I was rolling my eyes at the wrong time. Mind you, I loved the outfit, but my wife said my eyes told the truth and slammed the door as she walked out. Now along with this gift, I got the wonderful emotional gift that comes with some of these wonder drugs.

Mood or mental changes, including aggression, agitation, apathy, irritability, and mental depression. That is right. I was blessed with the aggression, irritability, and agitation. Suddenly my wife was living with a Jekyll and Hyde husband. This lasted about a year as we were on one of the last drugs we could try. One day, after a particularly exceptional display from husband Hyde, my wife packed her bags and said, enough is enough. I love you, however, I won't live with you like this. I'll come back after you get yourself under control. If that means you can't take any drugs, that will have to be your choice.

That event is what brought me to my doctor's office, on that sunny day back in 2009, to try and find something that would take care of this horrible mess, without side effects, so I could go back to living my life. That is when, after beseeching him for the cure for this so I could function again, he said those four nasty little words, "Nothing you can do!" I know my reaction to all of this and getting the medical divorce from him, was probably brought on by the drugs. It is his own fault because he prescribed them and never explained all the side effects that can have even more damaging effects than the neuropathy itself. Let me show you what I had to deal with. I'll just choose one of the drugs, that gave me several bouts of nasty side effects, to show you what I mean. This one is widely prescribed and I am sure many of you are using it without ever taking the time to read what it can do. You will see some of the effects I talked about earlier. Bear with me, this might take a few pages. Drug (name withheld to protect the innocent, me):

Major Side Effects

More common:

- Clumsiness or unsteadiness
- continuous, uncontrolled, back-and-forth, or rolling eye movements
- Aggressive behavior or other behavior problems
- anxiety
- concentration problems and change in school performance
- crying

- depression
- false sense of well-being
- hyperactivity or increase in body movements
- rapidly changing moods
- reacting too quickly, too emotional, or overreacting
- restlessness
- suspiciousness or distrust
- Fear

Less common:

- Black, tarry stools
- chest pain
- chills
- cough

- depression, irritability, or other mood or mental changes
- fever
- loss of memory
- pain or swelling in the arms or legs
- painful or difficult urination
- shortness of breath
- sore throat
- sores, ulcers, or white spots on the lips or in the mouth
- swollen glands
- unusual bleeding or bruising
- unusual tiredness or weakness

Incidence not known: FDA states that not all complaints are reported to them.

- Abdominal or stomach pain
- blistering, peeling, or loosening of the skin
- clay-colored stools
- coma
- confusion
- convulsions
- dark urine
- decreased urine output
- diarrhea
- dizziness
- fast or irregular heartbeat
- headache
- increased thirst

- itching or skin rash
- joint pain
- large, hive-like swelling on the face, eyelids, lips, tongue, throat, hands, legs, feet, or sex organs
- loss of appetite
- muscle ache or pain
- nausea
- red skin lesions, often with a purple center
- red, irritated eyes
- unpleasant breath odor
- vomiting of blood
- yellow eyes or skin

Minor Side Effects

More common:

- Blurred vision
- cold or flu-like symptoms
- delusions
- dementia
- hoarseness
- lack or loss of strength
- lower back or side pain
- swelling of the hands, feet, or lower legs
- trembling or shaking

Less common or rare:

- Accidental injury
- appetite increased
- back pain

- bloated or full feeling
- body aches or pain
- burning, dry, or itching eyes
- change in vision
- change in walking and balance
- clumsiness or unsteadiness
- congestion
- constipation
- cough producing mucus
- decrease in sexual desire or ability
- difficulty with breathing
- dryness of the mouth or throat
- earache
- excess air or gas in the stomach or intestines
- excessive tearing

- eye discharge
- feeling faint, dizzy, or lightheadedness
- feeling of warmth or heat
- flushed, dry skin
- flushing or redness of the skin, especially on the face and neck
- frequent urination
- fruit-like breath odor
- impaired vision
- incoordination
- increased hunger
- increased sensitivity to pain
- increased sensitivity to touch
- increased thirst
- indigestion

- noise in the ears
- pain, redness, rash, swelling, or bleeding where the skin is rubbed off
- passing gas
- redness or swelling in the ear
- redness, pain, swelling of the eye, eyelid, or inner lining of the eyelid
- runny nose
- sneezing
- sweating
- tender, swollen glands in the neck
- tightness in the chest
- tingling in the hands and feet
- trouble sleeping
- trouble swallowing

- trouble thinking

- twitching

- unexplained weight loss

- voice changes

- vomiting

- weakness or loss of strength

- weight gain

Can you believe it? This one little pill can cause so much harm, while supposedly doing good?

I guess I must be among both the common, and uncommon, people of this world. On this exploration of my options, I have found that I am not alone in this area. Many people have had the same, if not worse, experiences with their doctors, drugs, and neuropathy.

As I spent years following what I was told to do, I have also spent many years looking for relief, after my tantrum at my doctor's office. My exploration has taken thousands of dollars and many different treatments to get to one that finally worked. Here is where I leave you and let the creator of this treatment, tell her story. She is the reason I am walking free of pain, and was able to dance with my wife on our 25th wedding anniversary, and, I am now, barefoot again!

Chapter Three - They're Amputating My Foot!

These were the words spoken to me by a man, let's call him Mike, who walked through the door of my clinic one day, sat down and proceeded to cry. I asked if I could help him and he said, "A friend of mine is a client of yours, and he suggested I come see you." I asked him to explain what was going on. He said he was on his way to see his doctor for a final visit before they amputated his foot. I looked down at his swollen, blueish purple feet. He wore slippers due to the swelling. Mike explained that he had diabetes and that his feet were numb. A year earlier he had stepped on something and cut his foot. Due to the numbness, he didn't know he had, so it soon became infected. The doctor had tried everything and now the infection was into the bone. He wore an antibiotic pump and had for over six months. His doctor had scheduled an appointment to do one final test on his circulation, just to verify that it was inadequate, and, the reason his foot wouldn't heal.

He said, "I know I am not giving you much time to work with me, but, what do you think you would do?" I asked when his appointment was and he said he had an hour before he would have to leave. Luckily it was a day I wasn't busy. I couldn't do much, however, I had a new piece of medical equipment I decided to try. It had worked miracles on me and my circulation so I put it to the test, and put Mike on it. I had to keep it on low due to all the drugs in his body. I left him on it for 30 minutes, then sat him in a chair with his feet on a smaller version, on high, for the remainder of the hour. He thanked me and went to his appointment.

I went about my day and wondered how things went. I hoped he would stop back by and tell me. Well, just before closing for the day, he walked in with a big smile on his face. Look at my feet! I did and was surprised to see that the swelling was way down. He said, it was unbelievable! His doctor did the circulation test twice and couldn't believe it! His circulation was fine! He said they canceled his amputation and would continue with treatments for healing the wound.

This started my journey towards discovering a treatment for neuropathy that has helped improve the symptoms of all who have gone through my two-week therapy.

Chapter Four - The Pain is Unbearable

Not long after Mike came through my door, Steven came in with grief in his eyes. He said that he had heard through a friend that I might be able to help with his pain. He was from out of town and was hoping he could see me while he was here visiting. He explained that he was a scuba diver and had dived all over the world. Said he used to be very active. About 5 years earlier, as he was climbing up the ladder on the boat, he got a sharp pain in the arch of his foot. He said the pain was so unbearable that he fell back in the water and screamed. His companions thought something had attacked him. When he explained what had happened, they thought he got something in his foot, (they had walked on the ocean floor near coral). So, they carefully picked him out of the water and gingerly took his wetsuit off. Nothing there! They got a magnifying lens to check closer, however, there still was nothing showing. When he stood the pain was gone so he thought it was a freak incident.

When he got back home, he would occasionally get some shooting pains, that would almost bring him to his knees. He decided to see his doctor to find out what was going on. He was told that he was at the beginning stages of diabetic neuropathy. Steven had diabetes, and had for the last ten years. He hadn't heard of that before so he started doing some internet researches to learn more. He wasn't happy with what he found. As the years went by, the pain got so bad he couldn't scuba dive anymore. Trying to climb the ladder back into the boat, was too painful. He tried a slew of drugs over the years, with no lasting relief, just the side effects. Along with the deep pain, came the total foot numbness. He kept asking the doctor how it could hurt so bad yet he couldn't feel his foot? His doctor told him about the different areas; feet, hands, legs, and trunk, that it can affect. He said it shows up differently, yet the same, in many of his patients. Ironically, he found out that his doctor also had neuropathy. He was told that the only thing he could do was take the recommended course of drugs and join a support group. Steven believed his doctor, since he had been dealing with his own neuropathy for over 15 years. Of course, he would know all the options, wouldn't he? Every visit was five minutes about increasing one of his drugs or trying another. The remaining time was spent talking about fishing. This went on for years!

He said now it was to the point the it was extremely painful to walk barefoot from his bed to the bathroom. He said he had to have cushioned slippers on, all the time in the house and even in the shower. I told Steven that I was working on a treatment plan, that so far, (7 clients), had worked to improve the symptoms of neuropathy within two weeks. He said let's give it a try.

"I start everyone on a Monday and they come every day except weekends, for two weeks," I said. He said he would stay if it showed signs of working. We scheduled his appointments starting on the following Monday.

During the first week, his pain was significantly less. By the second Monday, he got up from my treatment table, and sat in a chair, to put his shoes on. He was looking at his feet and wiggling his toes. He asked, "Do you know the significance of this?" No, I said. He said, "I haven't been able to wiggle my toes in over five years!" I looked at him wiggling his toes, and I had to fight back the tears. "Do you know how good it feels to be able to go barefoot again, around my house and pool?" No, I said. He said "Walking around my house with my shoes off, is something I haven't been able to do in over five years! That is when I got tears in my eyes, at the miracle that was happening before me. Stevens words stayed in my mind for the rest of the afternoon as I thought about how fast this seemed to be working. By the end of the two weeks, Steven had full feeling in both feet, and the pain, when he would step on the handle of a broom, (simulating ladder rungs) was almost gone!

On the last day of his treatments, Steven had asked me if I knew of anything for Diabetes, that might help him. I told him that the only thing I recommend to my clients, outside of changes in their diet, is Syntra5. I gave him the information and told him to read it over before he decided. He looked at me with a quizzical expression, and asked, "Why?" I said so he could read the clinical research that shows its efficacy. Steven asked, "Do you think it works?" I said, "Yes, I have seen it work on all my clients that take is as directed on the label." He said, "Good enough for me!"

Over the next two months, Steven came in for a few more treatments, whenever he was in town and I had the time. His words, that day when he could wiggle his toes, were the inspiration for the name of my business and this book: "Barefoot Again."

I saw Steven about six months after his last treatment. He poked his head in my door one day, to see if I had a minute to talk. He wanted to share with me, his last doctors visit. He said his doctor did his normal diabetes testing along with his blood pressure and heart test and the works. Steven had a quadruple bypass about six years prior. He said his doctor said he needed to run a few tests again, as something must have gone wrong. Steven said, "My doctor told me that I must have completely changed my life because he couldn't detect any signs of diabetes." I told him, "Must be this stuff I'm taking from this gal that is a naturopath, homeopath or some kind of Path." (I'm none of those, by the way.) His doctor smirked and rolled his eyes. Steven said, "That was it for him." "I looked at him and said, well doc, not a damn thing you have given me over the years has worked!"

"And, just so you know, I quit taking all of them drugs you kept me on, six months ago." I laughed and said I was happy for him and his health. He said he had gone scuba diving with friends and that climbing out of the boat, he could feel pressure, but no pain!

Chapter Five - Haven't Felt My Feet in 20 Years

Do you know that feeling you get when someone walks into your life and you know that you will be changed forever? Well, that is what happened when Marlene came through my clinic door. Marlene has a quirky sense of humor and a heart of gold. She didn't however, have faith in anything working when it came to her neuropathy. She had lost the feeling in her feet over twenty years before, and it had slowly crept up her legs to about mid-calf. Even though she couldn't feel her feet, they had a sensation of always being hot. She slept with her feet out from under the covers and only wore sandals, even in winter. At night, she would get cramping up the inside of her legs so bad that she would have to get up and stand until they went away. This occurred at least four times a night, every night, for over twenty years. During those twenty years she had broken her ankle because she couldn't feel where she was placing her feet. She had stepped on things that cut her feet and created sores. Ones that needed operated on to clean out, all done without anesthesia or pain killer because she couldn't feel it. He toes would curl up backwards causing a hammertoe look. This caused the need for surgery to correct it, also done without any pain meds. Her story covered such a long period of time that during the course of her treatment, different things would pop into her head and she would add another incident to her case history.

Now the good news. By Wednesday of the first week of treatments, her cramping at night was significantly reduced. By Friday her feet weren't feeling as hot as usual. By the second Monday, she had almost complete feeling in her right foot and up her leg. All the nighttime cramping was gone. By the end of the two weeks of treatment, her left foot had about 75 percent feeling, she told me she actually had to pull her feet under the covers, because they felt cold! Also, while sitting on the couch, she pulled her foot away from her husband as he was rubbing them, because his hands felt cold! This was a miracle to me and to her! At the end of the two weeks of treatment, all the night time leg cramping was gone. We still didn't have complete feeling in her left foot and she felt some deep tightness in both feet. Marlene wanted to keep trying so decided to take a week off and then do another full week of treatments. We got rid of most of the tightness in both feet, however, the area where they had operated was still numb. She took another week off and then did a fourth full week of treatment. By the end of treatments, all the tightness was gone and a little more feeling came back in her left foot. However, due to the damage of the surgeries that were done on her wound, we were never able to get full feeling in her left foot. She has about a double silver dollar area that is still numb. She continued with a monthly maintenance treatment for about a year. She now comes for a maintenance treatment, whenever she feels she is backsliding. I see her about four times a year now for a maintenance treatment. Marlene was able to go on her first five-mile hike with her daughter last Fall. Didn't fall once, and, had stability and feeling all the way! She now tells me she loves me, every time I see her! This is priceless to me!

Chapter Six - What It's All About

I could go on and on with many stories, however, I think we need to talk about what I discovered and how I put my knowledge into practice. As you may remember from my bio, I also teach chemical safety. Now I know it seems quite different from the healing arts, however, I like learning many different things. I think every bit of knowledge we can gain, will help us in ways that we may not even understand, until we need it. That is what happened with me, when it came to working with my clients that had neuropathy. As I was filling out the intake paperwork and talking about what they had done for a living all their life, I realized that many of them had been in contact with different chemicals, be it by touch or by breathing, that can cause neuropathy. If I hadn't spent the time teaching students how to properly use protective equipment and clothing during handling of chemicals, I wouldn't have thought of this when dealing with neuropathy. I got a flash of one of the chemicals that I had given a class on, that if exposed to the skin, it could absorb in and one of the side effects could be neuropathy.

I started researching anything and everything that could chemically cause neuropathy in a person. I also researched how repeated exposure to small amounts could build up in the body and cause degradation of the nerves Myelin sheath, over time. This degradation leads to burning, tingling and numbness. I was shocked to see how many things can affect a person. Let me give you an example: A woman or man that has stayed home and worked all their life around the home, cleaning, taking care of the kids, (bath time), dishes, painting, new carpet, shampoo, spraying the weeds, you get my point, pretty much just living. The chemicals in many normal household cleaning agents, some even in soaps, can cause neuropathy. If you have a home with plywood, most do, then at 72 degrees, plywood can start off-gassing formaldehyde. Yes, you heard right, formaldehyde. One of Formaldehyde's side effects, from over exposure, can be neuropathy. This was evident with one of my clients that came to me with over eight years of neuropathy under his belt. "Nope, never touched or worked with chemicals." Arnold stated as I was questioning him during his intake. "Worked as a carpenter all my life and did a little wood working making cabinets." I asked if he was around plywood very much and he said, yes, every day. Turned out he owned his own business and kept a shop full of plywood and lumber. He spent many days in his shop building cabinets and refinishing old cabinets too. Just a fan, no air conditioner. Definitely over seventy-two degrees in the summer! I asked if he used much super glue in his cabinet building, and, he said he used a fair amount. Asked if he used any turpentine or wood strippers, paint thinners, wood stains, etc. You get my point, I am sure. Yes, he had worked around many chemicals, some unseen due to the nature of their use in construction, and others, that we tend to overlook, or, we don't take the time to read the labels, to determine what is a safe practice, when using them. All these chemicals build up in our system and can cause massive damage. Hence, damage to the Myelin Sheath surrounding the nerve, causing numbness, tingling, and burning.

Chapter Seven - What Does it all Mean?

Let me show you what I am talking about when it comes to nerve damage. Here you can see the difference between a normal cell, compressed cell, sheath loss, disconnection, and degeneration.

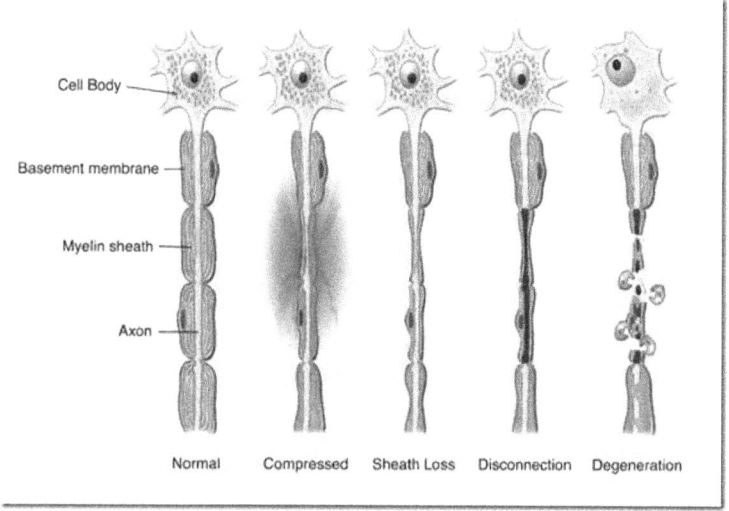

Accidents and injury can cause compression neuropathy. Certain chemicals can cause sheath loss. Sheath loss and accidents can cause disconnection and pretty much all of them can lead to degeneration.

Have you ever stopped to think about the word neuropathy? Well, if not, here it is. Neuropathy means nerve disease or damage. Symptoms can range from numbness or tingling, to pricking sensations or muscle weakness. Areas of the body may become abnormally sensitive leading to an exaggeratedly intense or distorted experience of touch. In such cases, pain may occur in response to a stimulus that does not normally provoke pain. Severe symptoms may include burning pain (especially at night), muscle wasting, paralysis, or organ or gland dysfunction. Damage to nerves that supply internal organs may impair digestion, sweating, sexual function, and urination. In the most extreme cases, breathing may become difficult, or organ failure may occur. It can involve much more than just your feet and hands. Peripheral Neuropathy is a condition that develops, as a result of damage to the peripheral nervous system. This is the vast communications network that transmits information between the central nervous system (the brain and spinal cord) and every other part of the body.

The Cleveland Clinic states: "It is estimated that about 25 to 30 percent of Americans will be affected by Neuropathy. Neuropathy occurs in 60 to 70 percent of people with diabetes."

With the current, 2017, US population, at only 25% that is 81,618,503 people with Neuropathy! That is a lot of suffering!

There are more than 100 types of peripheral neuropathies. Each has its own symptoms and prognosis. Peripheral neuropathy is neuropathy that affects the nerves of the extremities- the toes, feet, legs, fingers, hands, and arms. Some forms of neuropathy involve damage to only one nerve and are called mononeuropathies. More often, than not, multiple nerves are affected, called polyneuropathy. Some peripheral neuropathies are due to damage to the axons (the long, threadlike portion of the nerve cell), while others are due to damage to the myelin sheath, the fatty protein that coats and insulates the axon. Peripheral neuropathies may also be caused by a combination of both axonal damage and demyelination. Symptoms may be experienced over a period of days, weeks, or years.

Diabetes is the condition most commonly associated with neuropathy. The debilitating symptoms of peripheral neuropathy often seen in people with diabetes are sometimes referred to as diabetic neuropathy. The risk of having diabetic neuropathy rises with age and duration of diabetes. Neuropathy is most common in people who have had diabetes for decades and is usually more severe in those who have had difficulty controlling their diabetes, or those who are overweight or have elevated blood lipids and high blood pressure.

As a nutritional therapist, I understand the results of a poor diet. Peripheral neuropathy can occur as a result of malnutrition. Poor nutrition can be caused by an unbalanced diet and/or alcoholism. Additionally, a clear link has been established between a lack of vitamin B12 and peripheral neuropathy. Deficiencies of the vitamins B12 and folate as well as other B vitamins can cause damage to the nerves.

Have you ever felt like you are wearing gloves, when you aren't? How about socks, even though your feet are bare? This can be because of sensory nerve damage. Sensory nerve damage causes a variety of symptoms because sensory nerves have a broad range of functions. Larger sensory fibers enclosed in myelin, registers vibration, light touch, and position sense. Damage to large sensory fibers impairs touch, resulting in a general decrease in sensation. Since this is felt most in the hands and feet, people may feel as if they are wearing gloves and stockings even when they are not. This damage to larger sensory fibers may contribute to the loss of reflexes. Loss of your sense of position can make you unable to coordinate complex movements. These movements might seem like ordinary, everyday actions by our bodies, however, with the loss of position sense, movements like walking or fastening buttons, or to maintain your balance when your eyes are shut, suddenly becomes almost impossible.

Smaller sensory fibers without myelin sheaths transmit pain and temperature sensations. Damage to these fibers can interfere with the ability to feel pain or changes in temperature. People may fail to sense that they have been injured from a cut or that a wound is becoming infected. Loss of pain sensation is a particularly serious problem for people with diabetes. It is the number one factor contributing to the high rate of lower limb amputations among this population.

Other causes of neuropathy can be from disease, infection, toxins, medications, injury, and alcoholism. Some infections, including HIV/AIDS, Lyme disease, leprosy, and syphilis, can damage nerves. Post-herpetic neuralgia, a complication of shingles (varicella-zoster virus infection) is a form of neuropathy.

Alcoholism is often associated with peripheral neuropathy. Alcohol can do damage to the nerves by itself but most alcoholics, also suffer from poor nutrition. The alcohol along with the associated vitamin deficiencies that are common in alcoholics, can all lead to what is called Alcoholic Neuropathy.

Certain drugs and medications can cause nerve damage. Examples include cancer therapy drugs and antibiotics such as Metronidazole and Isoniazid.

Trauma or injury to nerves, including prolonged pressure on a nerve or group of nerves, is a common cause of neuropathy. Decreased blood flow (ischemia) to the nerves can also lead to long-term damage.

Environmental or industrial toxins such as lead, mercury, and arsenic can cause peripheral neuropathy. Other examples include, gold compounds, some industrial solvents, nitrous oxide, and organophosphate pesticides. Off-gassing (also known as out-gassing) refers to the release of airborne particulates or chemicals—dubbed volatile organic compounds (VOCs)—from common household products. In drafty old houses with lots of air changes it wasn't much of a problem, but as we build our houses tighter for energy efficiency, these chemicals can build up inside. The craziest part of it all is that we go out and buy these products, without knowing what's in them, and often stockpile them in the bathroom, the tiniest room of the house with the worst ventilation!

More VOC's! As I mentioned earlier, plywood in your house can also attribute to neuropathy. Judging by the words of the American Chemistry Council, Formaldehyde is positively benign, a natural part of our world. And it is, in small doses! Formaldehyde is a colorless chemical with a strong pickle-like odor that is commonly used in many manufacturing processes. It easily becomes a gas at room temperature, which makes it part of a larger group of chemicals known as volatile organic compounds (VOCs).

When an item gives off formaldehyde, it is released into the air through a process called off-gassing. It is a recognized carcinogen and causes eye and nose irritation. But, like I pointed out earlier, it can also cause neuropathy! Formaldehyde is a chemical used in the production of adhesives, bonding agents, and solvents. For this reason, it is commonly found in a variety of consumer products including: Pressed-wood products (plywood, particle board, paneling), foam insulation, wallpaper and paints, some synthetic fabrics (example: permanent press), some cosmetics and personal products.

Why is this so important to you? If you have been a carpenter, wood worker, carpet layer, painter, or a variety of other jobs, that use these products, you would then be able to better understand how you might have ended up with this disease.

New research, published in The Journal of the American Medical Association (JAMA), showed that certain acid reflux drugs are "significantly associated" with vitamin B12 deficiency. In turn, vitamin B12 deficiency causes serious health consequences including anemia, osteoporosis, depression, memory loss, dementia, neuropathy, and cardiovascular disease.

I spend quite a bit of time, on the subjects of possible exposure to toxins, and, nutritional assessment, with my clients. It helps me to identify the areas that may be lacking in their nutrition, and the forms of detoxification I will need to use, in treating my clients' neuropathy. If you have a chemical, sitting on the nerve, continuing to do damage, how can it heal?

Chapter Eight - Myths and My Opinion

Let me ask you a question. If you were to bind your hand tightly, in a position that it couldn't move for the entire day, every day, do you think you would lose the use of it? Of course, you would! Having people quit walking barefoot because it will harm them, is a myth to me. You can safely walk barefoot in your home, just make sure the way is clear. When I was in school for clinical foot therapy, my instructor talked about how bad hockey players feet are when they are done with their careers. He said, they shove their feet into shoes that are too small by about two sizes, so they won't slide. Their feet end up all bunched up and hideous looking. They hurt and sometimes it is hard for them to walk. He asked if we thought we could help get their feet back to normal. Of course, all of us said "No." "You're wrong!" "You can get them back to normal, it just takes work."

I realized that one of the biggest problems for people with neuropathy is that they keep their feet immobilized in their shoes. They tie them way to tight because they are afraid of slipping out of them, which just shuts more circulation off and makes the neuropathy spread faster. Yes, poor circulation is key to neuropathy's growth. It loves it when only a little blood is present. Wearing shoes too tight, also shuts down your lymphatic flow. Your lymphatic system, is the second circulatory system in your body. When your feet swell, it is because the lymphatic system is being either shut down, by constriction, or lack of movement. The only thing that moves the lymphatic flow, is the movement of your muscles and body. Yes, this includes the muscles and free movement, in your feet. Also, when you never walk around with your feet bare, your brain quits getting feedback, and hinders proper foot placement, so balance becomes an issue. You see, walking on the earth, absorbing the magnetic energy, is part of the human Biosystems. Now we have feet that are too weak to even walk barefoot on smooth floors. We used to be able to climb rocks, rubble, dirt, sticks, thorns and more. Now we must have a nice cushion on our soles.

Here are just a few of the benefits of walking barefoot for only 5 minutes a day. You can see improvement in:

Chronic muscle and joint pain along with other types of pain. Stress, Hypertension, PMS, Heart rate variability, Sleep disturbances including sleep apnea, Energy levels, Fasting glucose levels, Primary indications of osteoporosis, Asthmatic and respiratory conditions, Immune system activity and response, Arthritis and more. This is one of the reasons that I have all my clients walk barefoot, around their homes, during the two-week treatments. I know many of you will say that you are afraid of stepping on something and not knowing it. I say, pay attention to where you are placing your feet and check them when you sit down. You do want to be careful not to walk in an area that you could get a puncture wound. Just be careful where you place your feet and you will be fine. There is a new product that sticks to the soles of your feet, that will protect them from virtually all damage, including heat. It is in the development stage, and I will add it to the resource page, if available at time of printing.

For those of you that say my doctor won't let me go barefoot, I say, he isn't the one living with this, is he? Do you want to improve your situation? Then take the first step and let's get your feet moving again. You know when you are cutting up meat, the white stuff, between the muscles?

Sometimes it is thick and other times pretty thin. Well, that is called fascia. When you keep a muscle group from moving or limit its movement, this facia thickens. As time goes by, it hurts to move that area. This is why it might be painful, deep inside your feet, as you learn to walk barefoot again. You must break up all the facia, to get the smooth muscle action again. Your feet might also be too sensitive to touch, to even step on the floor barefoot. Give yourself some time on the BioMat and the NeurOil, before you try to walk barefoot. Do sit and wiggle your feet and toes as much as possible, with no shoes or socks on, and lightly touch them on the floor.

Chapter Nine - Where do you start?

The first step in treating peripheral neuropathy is to address any contributing causes such as infection, toxin exposure, medication-related toxicity, vitamin deficiencies, hormonal deficiencies, autoimmune disorders, or compression that can lead to neuropathy. Peripheral nerves can regenerate axons, as long as the nerve cell itself has not died, which may lead to functional recovery over time. Correcting an underlying condition often can result in the neuropathy resolving on its own as the nerves recover or regenerate.

Neuropathic pain, or pain caused by the injury to a nerve or nerves, is often difficult to control. This leads to most doctors treating their patients for "Pain Management." Unfortunately, some of these medications also carry a side effect of Neuropathy! Can you believe it? They are treating you for neuropathy with drugs that can cause neuropathy!

So, are medications the only answer? NO! There are other ways to address and help reduce or eliminate the symptoms of neuropathy.

In my clinic, I use ten different forms of therapy, combined into one treatment, as needed. However, the results you have heard about earlier in this book are from only seven forms of therapy, combined into one. I am always researching and adding new info to my therapies and will continue to do so. The results are life changing, to say the least.

Chapter Ten - The Light Bulb Comes On!

As I was sitting, listening to Ben talk about his wife and their dreams and plans for enjoying their retirement, it suddenly occurred to me that this treatment needed to be known to the world. I realized if I kept this to myself, and, only worked with my clients, the vast majority of neuropathy sufferers would never know about the options available to them. Now Ben is one of those fellows that sees the glass always full, no matter what, and finds something funny in almost every situation. He regaled me with stories of things he chose to find funny about his situation, from bouncing off the walls, literally, as he lost his balance to falling at his boss's feet. Said he had a few of those times while he was on leave from the service, he is a Marine, however it was caused usually by first enjoying a few libations. He told me of one day being called into his boss's office, not for anything bad, well, that was until he lost his balance and fell at his boss's feet! All he could think about was joking about a raise. So, in Ben fashion, he said, "Please, please, can I have a raise?" Luckily at this point his boss knew about the imbalance problems and the drugs that added to it. He laughed and said," NOPE! But, good try none the less!" Now Ben's story is just one of millions. The thought of how difficult this truly is, and how humiliating many situations are, that can arise around everyday dealings with this horrible disease, brought tears to my eyes. I thought of all the suffering going on, with no real hope. I want you to know, there is hope! Even if you can't make it to my clinic, at this time, there is a lot you can do at home to get some relief and improve the symptoms of neuropathy. In the not too distant future, I will be adding more places to go for treatments. Many treatment and training centers are planned in Countries around the World.

I will explain, in detail, part of the treatment that I perform at the clinic. I will also let you know what you can do at home for yourself. You will find a resource area at the back of this book for everything you are going to learn about. Don't worry, this won't take a degree in science to understand. Ben said to explain it, in easy to understand terms, just like I did for him.

My clients come in for a consultation, prior to beginning the treatment. We fill out a 10-page intake together, one that I developed over the years. This gives me a clear picture of what I will use to treat their individual needs and what needs to be detoxed from their system or their subconscious. Yes, I do have some clients that are suffering from PTSD or extreme high stress, that need the mind and subconscious detoxed. This is done with hidden belief and emotion release, along with energy healing. That is a whole other book. You will find it listed in the resource section.

During the initial intake and consult, clients will receive a set of instructions (feel free to tear out this page in the resource section), on what they need to eliminate from their diet and things they should add. I then set up a two-week treatment plan that is customized for each client. Clients are sent home with the Detoxi Salts and any supplements that they will need to take before coming to therapy. All therapies are pretty much the same, with just a little tweaking to customize it to individual needs. A client comes Monday through Friday for two weeks. This is the jump start program and most people only need to come in for maintenance therapy after that. I am going to give you a little sense of how it goes:

Monday ~ I map the feet and lower legs for sensitivity to extremely light pressure. Think, touch of a feather. Then I map them for moderate to deep pressure. Is it sore, numb or a feeling of tightness? After the mapping is done, so we can track progress, I place their feet in a foot soak that I formulated for detoxing from many different chemicals known to cause neuropathy. It also helps loosen the muscles of the feet, which is vital for the first massage. Now this isn't one of those foot soaks that you look at and go, wow, look at all that junk in the water! Most chemicals are so minute, you would not be able to see them with the naked eye. Think of breathing the chemical, formaldehyde, from the off-gassing of plywood. Do you think it would come out of your cells as a particle that could be seen, when it went into your body as air? I am not saying that some of those machines that claim to pull junk out of your feet, don't work. However, our skin looks like tiny balls floating on the surface of water. The interstitial fluid surrounding all our skin cells is what holds some of the waste and toxins in our body. What comes out of it, can't be larger than what can squeeze through the framework of our cells. Just saying,' I don't see it happening. However, the color of the water can change.

After the foot soak, my client lays down on my treatment table. The table has a BioMat that is an FDA approved medical device for pain and stress. Recently approved for arthritis specific pain also.

This mat is much more than just a mat! It won a Grand Prize in 2010, in the Medical Device Field from the Royal Swedish Academy of Science. The technology comes from the Scientist at NASA. They use this form of technology to help the astronauts when they go into outer space. I don't want to get too technical, but at the same time, I want to give you an idea of what this amazing piece of medical equipment is.

The BioMat is a "pad" which lies on top of a massage table. It converts electricity through an Electromagnetic Interceptor, which then converts it into Far Infrared Rays (FIR), and Negative Ions. Negative Ions and Far Infrared Rays, are transferred through Amethyst Quartz Crystals, which cover the entire surface of the BioMat. Amethyst produces naturally occurring far infrared waves. These frequencies penetrate 6 inches deep into the body, stimulating the healing process. I also lay a mini-BioMat on top of my clients as they rest. When you are "sandwiched" between the large and small BioMats, this translates into healing frequencies penetrating 12 inches deep within the body. This Supports the Immune System and aides the body in reducing inflammation, increases blood flow and tissue oxygenation and promotes relaxation. This accelerates and deepens all healing processes.

You will also be on a Quantum Energy Pad. This is another form of energy that effects the cells of the body in a positive way. Quantum energy helps in the stability of Brain Waves as the pad reduces Beta waves, seen in stressful situations, while increasing Alpha waves creating a state of relaxation and allowing for refreshing sleep and vitality. It also helps promote blood circulation and enhances resistance against harmful germs and bacteria.

I created a Therapeutic Essential oil blend that has over 31 different oils in it. These oils are based on ones that will help with detox, nerve stimulation, relaxation and much more. I massage this oil into the feet and up the legs to the knees. Most therapeutic essential oil blends, are mix with a ratio of about 1 drop to every 10 to 20 drops or more of carrier oil. I mix mine in a 1:1 ratio and only use a carrier oil that also is good for nerve health. After I massage this in, I then perform a form of massage that consists of tiny motions, over the entire foot and up the leg to the knee. I won't go into detail as to what I am talking about or "looking for" with my fingers, I will leave that for my students.

After the massage, I have my client pull their feet up and I place the mini mat over the top of their feet. They relax as the massage oil, amplified by the long wave Far-Infrared and negative ions, penetrate deep within to help promote healing. Depending upon the situation, I will use either Reiki, Chakra balancing or audible healing frequencies to help promote healing, or a combination of all.

This is a typical treatment day; however, they change according to what is needed. All in all, it is a very pleasant experience! Most of my clients tell me that they miss coming in every day. Some will even add another week, even though they already feel their feet, just to make sure they get even more benefit. I think it is because they miss all the daily attention, or maybe me!

Chapter Eleven - At Home, On Your Own

The thought of being alone in this, might sound scary or impossible to you right now, but don't worry, it isn't. Taking care of yourself at home, is actually quite simple. First off let's go over what you need to work on yourself at home. Then we will cover what you need to eliminate from your diet, and what you need to add to it. I will explain why you need to do these things. I do understand that money is an issue for many people so I am going to go with the items in order of priority. For those that can afford it, I use #1, 2, 3, and 7 for each client, during the two-week treatment. As far as the supplements go, it depends upon what I learn about each client, during the intake process. Some people have been on a cleansing process and they don't need the Detox foot soak. Some are already taking the Juice Plus+ and have corrected their diet. What you choose to take, will depend upon how you have been feeding and caring for your body. For at home use, I have listed items in order of priority, if on a budget:

Mini-BioMat ~ #1

DETOXi Salts ~ #2

Barefoot Again NeurOil ~ #3

Juice Plus+ ~ #4

Barefoot Again, Detox Foot Soak ~ #5

Barefoot Again, Restore Foot Soak ~ #6

One bed size BioMat ~ # 7

NanoEnhanced Hemp Oil ~ may be added at any time: Legal in all 50 States. Learn more about it on my website.

Neuroveen ~ May be added at any time.

You will use the Mini BioMat at least twice a day, by placing your feet on it or bending it over your feet, like a taco, while you read, watch TV or when you are on your computer. You can sit all day with it on low, this just depends on your activity level. Start on the lowest setting and work your way up to the high. Use for at least 30 minutes, twice a day. Be sure to move your feet around to different areas of the mat, to keep them from getting too hot in one area. You might need to check the temperature with your hands, dependent upon your ability to feel heat, and the level of numbness in your feet. Now, for the one on your bed, when you sleep at night, keep in on the low setting. I have a cartoon manual on my BioMat website that is fun and informative on how to use the BioMats properly. It is loaded with great information. Depending upon the prescriptions you are taking, you can increase the heat level as you wish. I have added the contraindications in the resource area of this book. Please read before using the BioMat. Remember, this is NOT a heating pad, this is a medical device! It generates a different form of heat and does not get warm until you place your body on it or it has something to bounce the infrared off.

Drink plenty of water! Most clients tell me that they drink LOTS of water. However, when I tell them that they need half their bodyweight in ounces a day, I get the Lucy Look! You know the one, Big Eyes, looking at me like I am crazy! OK, 'I Love Lucy' was one of my favorite shows on TV, so, that is what I think of, when they are glaring at me like I need to be committed! You see, your cells need water to function properly. Think of running your car on only half the oil it needs to lubricate everything, or, trying to cook pancakes by making the batter with half the fluid necessary for it to pour out. Did you know that just drinking enough water a day can lower your blood pressure? Cheap too! If your blood gets too thick, which it does when it doesn't have enough water, then it takes more pressure to move it throughout your body. I have had clients tell me that by just continuing that one thing past the two weeks of therapy, their blood pressure is lower. So as an example: if you weigh 175 pounds you would divide that by 2 = 87.5 ounces of water. I have my clients get a 20-ounce bottle, stainless steel, glass, or hard plastic and fill it up with good spring water or well water, not city water or individually bottled water. The plastic bottles that are basically disposable, leach chemicals from the plastic into the water, that can build up in your cells and cause damage. During my Nutritional Therapy training, we were told of a study done in Europe, where they biopsied the abdominal fat of 1500 women, to try and determine why, even though they exercised, ate healthy and drank plenty of water, they still had excess stomach fat. What they found was astounding! There were chemicals found in their fat cells, that came from the plastic of the drinking bottles, that the women were consuming every day. You see, the way the body works when you consume something is like this. Digestion starts in your mouth. The minute a food or drink hits your tongue, the process begins. It is identified so your body knows how to use it. If it is a chemical, it knows that it can't be used as a building block for your body, so it wraps it in a protective layer of fat and stores it. You see, your body is trying to protect you from yourself! In order to get your water down, you can add fresh squeezed lemon, lime or orange, make herbal tea (no caffeinated tea), get a watermelon and whiz it up in the blender with water, add peppermint leaves, whatever you need to do to get your water intake for the day. So, go ahead and add some flavor, as long as it is organic, and, not one of the premade water enhancers. Again, we are trying to get rid of all the chemicals in your body, not add to them. Watermelon juice, made in a blender, is a great detoxing drink. Melons are considered an almost completely predigested food, because the nutrient from them is almost instantly accessible to the body. I go through about one large watermelon a week, this way.

I'm going to divert a little here, and let Mike talk about using the BioMat at home. It really isn't hard to do. It is the foundation of getting your best results. Mike agreed to let me work with him to test the results of using just the BioMat, on his neuropathy. I will say it was hard to NOT do the complete treatment, knowing I would get the best results if I did. But, research is imperative to any treatment. So, I will let Mike tell you what he experienced during this test of the BioMat.

In Mike's Words:

My Neuropathy

My name is Mike McDonald, I'm 81 years old and my wife and I live in Roseville, Ca. The following is my experience with Neuropathy. The date is mid-August 2017.

About a month ago I was wrapping up some acupuncture treatments and mentioned to my acupuncturist that I was having problems with my neuropathy relative to losing my balance. I've had neuropathy for four or five years and I lost maybe a third of my feeling up to my ankles, with very little change for several years. I thought I was doing just fine until the balance issue showed up and made it much more serious. My acupuncturist gave me a business card for a person named Roxanne DeLillo, who does neuropathy treatments and she was in the same building. My Neurologist told me that neuropathy can't be cured. However, I have a tendency to believe in holistic medicine and decided to give Roxanne a call.

I called her the next day and told her that my wife and I had very limited resources due to the fact that we never recovered from the 2008 housing crash just like millions of retired middle class. She was very easy to talk to and I felt we would really hit it off. We discussed the cost and it was something we could not handle. She then told me that she always wondered how much the BioMat by itself, contributed to the results she got from the complete treatment. Apparently, she uses the BioMat plus seven other techniques, and she has never failed to improve the symptoms of neuropathy in all her clients. Then she made me an offer I couldn't refuse. She suggested I volunteer to use the BioMat only, at no cost to me, so she could determine how much it contributed to her neuropathy program, and how much improvement it might give on its own. I almost jumped through the phone saying YES. This would involve ten 1/2-hour treatments excluding weekends.

After the 1st treatment my toes felt more normal. During the next three or four treatments, my balance had completely returned. which was a huge relief. After the ten treatments,

I believe I had 90% of my feeling back which may be as good as it gets at 81 years old.

My wife and I will be forever in Roxanne's debt. I had a feeling that she did not want to let me go until she figured out a way to help me. She is an unbelievable and caring holistic healer.

Chapter Twelve – Get the Gunk Out

When dealing with neuropathy, you must think about it on a cellular level. When a cell is overloaded with wastes from years of toxic substances, it cannot perform correctly. This is the next step in cleaning out the gunk that has built up, and breathing new life into a cell. I use Richway's DETOXi Salts for this, along with the BioMat. The DETOXi Salts are to be used as directed. The primary benefits of DETOXi include cleansing the bodies organs and balancing the cells osmosis pressure bringing noticeable improvement to your energy levels and stamina.

A cell also needs energy to function correctly. The one thing that I have noticed with almost all my clients, is that they really haven't eaten well over the years. Now this isn't just the diabetic clients, this is almost everyone, including a dietician. Sometimes we don't practice what we preach! Over the years I have had many different supplements given to me and pushed on me by people in the know, and those that think they know. As an Internationally Trained Nutritional Therapist, I tend to listen to what I believe is true and what science has proven. I only recommend one product, and I am also a user of this product for over 10 years. It is backed by numerous independent studies by universities and hospitals. It is Juice Plus+, not to be confused with other juice products. It is in capsule form, not a juice. More than 30 Juice Plus+ Research studies have been conducted in leading hospitals and universities around the world, including:

- Academic Centre for Dentistry Amsterdam, The Netherlands
- Brigham Young University
- Charité University Medical Centre, Berlin, Germany
- Georgetown University
- Kings College in London
- Medical University of Graz, Austria
- Medical University of Vienna
- Nemours Children's Clinic

- Tokyo Women's Medical University, Japan
- University of Arizona
- University of Birmingham, England
- University of Florida
- University of Maryland School of Medicine
- University of Milan, Italy
- University of Mississippi Medical Center
- University of North Carolina-Greensboro
- University of South Carolina
- University of Sydney in Australia
- University of Texas Health Science Center
- University of Texas/MD Anderson
- University of Witten-Herdecke, Germany
- University of Würzburg, Germany
- Vanderbilt University

- Wake Forest University funded by the National Cancer Institute
- Yale University-Griffin Hospital Prevention Research Center

I have seen the beneficial results of proper nutrition on disease of all kinds. From neuropathy to PTSD, your body needs the proper fuel, the nutritional balance of nature, to work correctly. Think of it as the premium fuel for your cells. One surgical client of mine, at an aftercare I used to run, had over 18 inches of his spine fused. He spent a month at my place, and, during that time and two weeks prior to his surgery, he started taking double the daily dose of Juice Plus+. When I took him into his first checkup appointment, he walked in from the parking lot. His surgeon looked at him and said, "Wow, I have never had anyone walk into my office on their first appointment, after that surgery!" That was a big eye opener for me. I knew it worked, I read all the science, I mean ALL of it, because I am a science nut, but this was a close to home moment. I had complete bloodwork done on me before I started using it, just to see if it really would get in and do what it said it would. I know, I read the science, but, I still wanted to know what it did for me. I took it for four months, that is what it takes for many cells to change over in the body, then had my blood tested again. The change was amazing! My doctor said she needed to do it herself. That is what started me using it in all my therapies. One neuropathy client swears by it. Said it helped with the pain and many of the symptoms, even before coming to see me. So, I always recommend it to all my clients. Of course, you will take it as directed on the bottle.

The Detox foot soak is to be used once a week. You will use it at home differently than what I use it at the clinic. Since you won't be massaging your feet, you will use it at the end of each week for a month. You will use the Restore foot soak at the beginning of each week, for a month.

The NeurOil, should be used twice a day, on clean feet. It is imperative that your feet are free of dirt and lotions. Massage in as best you can, for as long as you can. Massage is very beneficial for the neuropathic foot.

If you want help with the symptoms of neuropathy while going through this self-care treatment, Neuroveen is wonderful! Many of my clients continue to take it even after they have feeling back. They say it just makes them feel better, kind of like a safety net. It is not considered a cure, but it does help with the symptoms.

You will also want to reengage your brain. You can do this by focusing on each part of your foot, toes to heel, and lightly rubbing them across the floor or something soft, while you look at them. This helps the brain reconnect after being shut off from the sense of touch for so long. It is critical that you do this every day. I once had a client that kept saying she couldn't feel anything, however, she would jerk her foot or twitch when I touched certain areas. I told her that I wanted her to really think about it and see if she could feel anything. She kept saying no. So, I got specific. I asked her if she felt me touching her toe? She said yes. I said "OK", how about here? She said yes. I then told her I wanted her to pay closer attention because she was beginning to feel, but, her brain had not accepted the fact yet. To do this she had to sit and do the exercise I explained, and I had her watch me touch areas of her feet to make the visual connection. She is the lady that couldn't feel her feet for over twenty years.

Chapter Thirteen – Changing for the Better

You've made it this far, don't give up! Here are 16 "lifestyle" recommendations for anyone serious about their health and getting over Neuropathy. If you make these changes in your everyday activity, you will see and feel positive changes in your health. These will be in the resource section, without the explanation. Easier to put on your refrigerator!

Restrictions

- ❖ Don't drink soda (regular/diet), but especially diet! Ever. Well, except maybe a few times a year in a Root Beer float, with real sugar. I'm not a tyrant! Really! This leniency in your diet, is not to be abused though.

- ❖ Extremely Limit refined sugar intake. I don't allow any during the two-week therapy. We all know what these are: cookies, cake, candy, ice cream, etc. There is no place in a healthy person's life for these nonfoods.
- ❖ Don't eat fried or deep-fried foods. These "foods" are perhaps the most damaging of any in the long-run. Researchers at Scripps Research Institute in Florida, say that fast food, aside from being the 'convenient option' for sedentary lifestyles of most Americans today, is as addictive as cigarette smoking and heroin.

- No processed meats. According to the World Health Organization, Bacon, ham and sausages rank alongside cigarettes as a major cause of cancer, this places cured and processed meats in the same category as asbestos, alcohol, arsenic and tobacco.

- Don't drink milk and limit fruit juice. Commercial milk is not fit for consumption by humans. Yes, I know all of you that grew up with milk at every meal will argue over this one. For one reason, cow's milk is full of hormones that were meant to feed a calf and make it grow and get strong, fast. Don't drink it. Well, maybe every once in a while, when you have a Starbucks, but, not more than once a month.

Fruit juice, unless you are blending the whole fruit in a Vitamix or blender, with water, also needs to be limited, as it is high in sugar, and you need the fiber that comes with the whole food.

- ❖ Limit consumption of grain-based foods (bread, cereal, pasta). Grains are stored in Cilos with insecticide. Did you know that gluten intolerance didn't even exist up until about the 1960's but mostly started in the 1970's? (I'm not talking about Celiac disease, I'm talking about gluten intolerance). That is when our grain started being stored with Aluminum Phosphide to protect it from Weevil infestation. When it comes out of the bins to be ground, that chemical residue is still on the wheat and is then ground into flour. If you are wondering how bad this chemical is, let me tell you. According to my HAZMAT books (I teach hazardous materials handling and cleanup operations), it is a deadly poison and dangerous when it is wet! You most likely don't have an allergic reaction to wheat, you have an allergic reaction to Aluminum phosphide and several other insecticides that have built up an intolerance in your body. Some of these chemicals can also cause neuropathy. Here are some of the chemicals that are used in the storage of our grain supplies in the US. Actellicm Aluminum phosphide, Centynal. Diacon IGR, Prozap Insect Guard, Dipel and other Bt products, Profume, Pyganic, Evergreen,

Pyronyl and other pyrethrin products, Storcide II. These are just a few of them and are used on corn, wheat, barley, oats, peanuts, popcorn, soybeans, sorghum and rye. This is why I tell you to eliminate some of these from your diet. I use Ezekiel Bread or a bread that states it is non-GMO, Organic, and chemical free.

- ❖ Eat whole fruit (three small servings/day). Eat more vegetables than fruit. Any phytonutrients found in whole fruit can be found in vegetables without excess carbohydrates. I am not a fanatic about limiting whole fruit. When you are craving fruit, eat it! Unless you are diabetic and can't handle the sugar.

- ❖ Drink half your body weight in ounces of water a day. Only pure spring water or well water if you have good water, not water in a small plastic bottle or city water.

- ❖ Eat only good Himalayan salt or an equally good sea salt. Get rid of any table salt! Salt itself is not bad. A body needs 1 – 1 ½ teaspoons of pure salt a day to clean out the waste in our cells. DETOXi Salts help with the cleanup but I prefer Himalayan for my food.

Additions

Add these to your diet, daily.

- ❖ Eat vegetables with every meal if possible. Eat raw as much as you can. Concentrate on the dark, leafy greens and other colorful vegetables.

- Eat healthy fats every day. These are: flax meal/oil, organic coconut oil, borage oil, extra virgin olive oil. Eat these raw, not cooked.
- Eat some protein with every meal. Breakfast should be predominately protein and healthy fats. Primary protein sources are: meats, beans, nuts, cheeses, and eggs.
- Eat 3-5 small meals/day. Eat your last meal of the day at least four hours before bedtime.
- Get fit. Our bodies are designed to work and sweat. There is simply no substitute for exercise. Get as close to your ideal weight/height ratio as possible.
- Take Juice Plus+ to bridge the gaps in your nutrition.

❖ Take a good probiotic, I recommend Custom Probiotics. You need 400 - 700 billion, per day, to reset the function of your gut. Custom Probiotics has formulated an 11 strain Probiotic powder. It has 260 billion cfu's /gram. That is about the size of a ¼ tsp. I love this probiotic! And yes, you read that right, billions, not millions. You can't take a million-man army against a trillion-man army, and expect to win. The same is true of your gut. It is a war for your health in there! A little trivia for you. Did you know that within the human gastrointestinal microbiota, (your gut) exists a complex ecosystem of approximately 300 to 500 bacterial species, comprising nearly 2 million genes (the microbiome)? Indeed, the number of bacteria, within the gut, is approximately 10 times that of all of the cells in the human body, and the collective bacterial genome is vastly greater than the human genome.

- ❖ If you are a diabetic, I recommend Syntra5. I have seen it work wonders on my clients. It has over a million dollars in clinical studies. It has been shown to drop your A1c, faster than any drug on the market today.

Making these changes in your life, will bring rewards that you can now only imagine. This is the only life we have, so treat it like it's the most valuable thing in the world. It is! Remember, you must be the one to change your health, not your doctor, not me, not your spouse, you!

Chapter Fourteen – You Can Do This!

So, there you have it! I have shown you all the things you can do at home, to help improve your symptoms of neuropathy. If you don't feel like going it alone, you can contact me for information on therapists in your area, or come to my clinic in Roseville, CA. I also do phone consultations (if time is available) to help you figure out what direction is best for you.

I hope this has helped take some of the mystery out of neuropathy and will help you take control of your own path ahead. I do believe that everyone can benefit from this in one way or another.

Remember, slow circulation is the power behind neuropathy. The less circulation, the faster it can spread!

Enjoy your journey and congratulations on taking this step towards walking Barefoot Again!

Resources, Routines & Restrictions

For all of you that would rather have one spot to go for this info, go to:

www.barefoot-again.com/resources.

Everything below is listed on the Resource page.

NeurOil, Barefoot Again Detox and Restore, foot soaks, are all available through the above link.

BioMat: https://dakotarox.thebiomatcompany.com

Juice Plus+: http://rdelillo.juiceplus.com

NanoEnhanced Hemp Oil:

http://rdelillo.primemybody.com

Neuroveen: www.hellolife.com

Custom Probiotics, 11 Strain:

http://www.customprobiotics.com

Amicus Meus ~ 91 Hours to an Extraordinary Life! This is my book on releasing negative beliefs, emotions and more. You will find it on Amazon, and at Barnes & Nobel's.

Changing your routine

Here are your lifestyle recommendations for improving your Neuropathy and Diabetes. If you make these changes in your everyday activity, you will see and feel dramatic positive changes in your health.

Restrictions

- Don't drink soda (regular/diet).
- Limit refined sugar intake. We all know what these are: cookies, cake, candy, ice cream, etc.
- Don't eat fried or deep-fried foods. These "foods" are the most damaging of any in the long-run.
- Don't drink milk and limit fruit juice.
- Limit consumption of grain-based foods (bread, cereal, pasta).
- Eat whole fruit (three servings/day). Eat more vegetables than fruit.
- Drink half your body weight in ounces of water a day. Only pure spring water or well water, not in a small plastic bottle.

❖ Eat only good Himalayan salt. Get rid of any table salt! A body needs 1 – 1 ½ teaspoons of pure salt a day to clean out the waste in our cells.

Additions

- Eat vegetables with every meal. Eat raw as much as you can. Concentrate on the dark, leafy greens and other colorful vegetables.
- Eat healthy fats every day. These are: flax meal/oil, organic coconut oil, borage oil, fish oils, extra virgin olive oil. Eat these raw, not cooked.
- Eat some protein with every meal. Breakfast should be predominately protein and healthy fats. Primary protein sources are: meats, beans, nuts, cheeses, and eggs.
- Eat 3-5 small meals/day. Try to eat your last meal of the day at least three hours before bedtime.

❖ Get fit. Our bodies are designed to work and sweat. There is simply no substitute for exercise. Get as close to your ideal weight/height ratio as possible.

❖ Take Syntra5 if you have diabetes and Juice Plus+ to bridge the gaps in your nutrition. Take Custom Probiotics 11 Strain formula. It is simply the best way to get your gut back to functioning the way it should.

Making these changes in your life will bring rewards that you can now only imagine. This is the only life we have, so treat it like it's the most valuable thing in the world. It is. Remember, your health is counting on you to make good decisions.

Avoiding the Everyday Toxins

Here are several toxins that we encounter on a daily basis. These toxins accumulate in your body and cause many diseases. Read your labels and avoid them at all costs!

Coal Tar: A known carcinogen banned in the EU, but still used in North America. Used in dry skin treatments, anti-lice and anti-dandruff shampoos, also listed as a color plus number, i.e. FD&C Red No. 6.

DEA/TEA/MEA: Suspected carcinogens used as emulsifiers and foaming agents for shampoos, body washes, soaps.

Ethoxylated surfactants and 1,4-dioxane: Never listed because it's a by-product made from adding carcinogenic ethylene oxide to make other chemicals less harsh. The Environmental Working Group (EWG) has found 1,4-dioxane in 57 percent of baby washes in the U.S. Avoid any ingredients containing the letters "eth."

Formaldehyde: Probable carcinogen and irritant found in nail products, hair dye, fake eyelash adhesives, shampoos. Banned in the EU.

Fragrance/Parfum: A catchall for hidden chemicals, such as phthalates. Fragrance is connected to headaches, dizziness, asthma, and allergies.

Hydroquinone: Used for lightening skin. Banned in the UK, rated most toxic on the EWG's Skin Deep database, and linked to cancer and reproductive toxicity.

Lead: Known carcinogen found in lipstick and hair dye, but never listed because it's a contaminant, not an ingredient.

Mercury: Known allergen that impairs brain development. Found in mascara and some eyedrops.

Mineral oil: By-product of petroleum that's used in baby oil, moisturizers, styling gels. It creates a film that impairs the skin's ability to release toxins.

Oxybenzone: Active ingredient in chemical sunscreens that accumulates in fatty tissues and is linked to allergies, hormone disruption, cellular damage, low birth weight.

Parabens: Used as preservatives, found in many products. Linked to cancer, endocrine disruption, reproductive toxicity.

Paraphenylenediamine (PPD): Used in hair products and dyes, but toxic to skin and immune system.

Phthalates: Plasticizers banned in the EU and California in children's toys, but present in many fragrances, perfumes, deodorants, lotions. Linked to endocrine disruption, liver/kidney/lung damage, cancer.

Placental extract: Used in some skin and hair products, but linked to endocrine disruption.

Polyethylene glycol (PEG): Penetration enhancer used in many products, it's often contaminated with 1,4-dioxane and ethylene oxide, both known carcinogens.

Silicone-derived emollients: Used to make a product feel soft, these don't biodegrade, and also prevent skin from breathing. Linked to tumor growth and skin irritation.

Sodium lauryl (ether) sulfate (SLS, SLES): A former industrial degreaser now used to make soap foamy, it's absorbed into the body and irritates skin.

Talc: Similar to asbestos in composition, it's found in baby powder, eye shadow, blush, deodorant. Linked to ovarian cancer and respiratory problems.

Toluene: Known to disrupt the immune and endocrine systems, and fetal development, it's used in nail and hair products. Often hidden under fragrance.

Triclosan: Found in antibacterial products, hand sanitizers, and deodorants, it is linked to cancer and endocrine disruption. Avoid the brand Microban. Reading the labels on everything needs to become a habit. All of these toxins can do damage to the cells in your body. Pay close attention to what you put on your skin, breath in (as in air fresheners) or take into your mouth.

Contraindications

Here is a list of Contraindications for the large (bed size) BioMat. Using the Mini Mat on your feet should be fine, unless you are an organ transplant recipient. You will then need to consult with your doctor before using the BioMat, however, it is always recommended to consult with your physician before the use of the BioMat.

***Remember to stay hydrated while using the BioMat.

Contraindications as stated by Richway:

Organ Transplants -

Recipients who have had any type of organ transplant (Kidney, Heart, Liver, etc) **should not** use the Biomat. After an organ transplant, patients will need to take immunosuppressant (anti-rejection) drugs to help prevent their immune system from attacking, or rejecting, the new organ. The use of the Biomat's Far Infrared Rays increases immune system function, which will tell your body to attack the new organ.

External Pacemaker –

We recommend anyone who uses an external pacemaker that they **should not** use the Biomat.

Renal or Kidney Failure –

We recommend anyone who has Renal or Kidney failure that they **should not** use the Biomat. The use of the Biomat increases circulation of the blood, which may increase the blood flow to the kidneys causing stress.

Use with Caution:

Heat Sensitive MS –

We recommend anyone with Heat Sensitive MS to use the Biomat with **no heat and negative ions only**. Anyone with other types of MS can use the Biomat at any setting.

Radiation Therapy/Chemotherapy –

We recommend anyone that has currently received radiation treatments or chemotherapy to use the Biomat with **negative ions only**. **Consult your physician** before using the Biomat with any heat settings.

Brain Tumor –

We recommend anyone with a brain tumor to use the Biomat on **low heat only** (95F-113F).

Bypass Surgery –

We recommend anyone who has undergone bypass surgery to use the Biomat on **low heat only** (95F-113F). The use of the Biomat increases circulation of the blood, which can cause normal blood vessels to expand. Some people who have gone through bypass surgery, experience discomfort since their blood vessels can't expand.

Internal Pacemaker–

We recommend anyone who uses a pacemaker to use the Biomat on **low heat only** (95F-113F). The use of the Biomat increases circulation of the blood, which can cause an increase in heartbeat. Some people who use a pacemaker, experience discomfort since their heart beat is being controlled.

Diabetics –

We recommend anyone with Diabetes to use the Biomat on **low heat only** (95F-113F). Diabetics' skin is weak, which can cause low heatburn from the use of the Biomat. Once the skin is damaged, it may be difficult to recover

High Blood Pressure (Hypertension) –

We recommend people with chronically high blood pressure (hypertension) to use the Biomat with caution before and after use, and on **low heat only** (95F-113F). Sudden changes in body temperature and/or weather temperature may cause an increase in blood pressure.

Newborn Babies –

We recommend parents with newborns to wait until their baby is at least 6 months old before using the Biomat on **low heat only (95F-104F)** or **negative ions only**.

Infants –

We recommend that infants using the Biomat should use it on **low heat only** (95F-113F) and with adult supervision. If temperature is too high for the child, the temperature can't be controlled without an adult. Please use with caution.

Pregnancy –

We recommend women in their pregnancy to use the Biomat on **low to medium heat** (95F-131F).

Surgical Implants –

Recipients of Titanium, Metal, Ceramic, or Plastic implants can use the Biomat. Surgical implants generally reflect infrared rays and are not heated by an infrared heat system. Anyone who experiences pain in those areas should check with their physician.

Silicon - Silicon implants may be warmed by infrared rays. Silicon is known to melt at over 200 degrees Celsius / 392 Fahrenheit, so it should not be adversely affected by infrared rays. It is advised that you consult your surgeon before use.

Pain:

Pain should not be experienced when using the Biomat. However, the infrared heat will go to areas of disease or discomfort so some people may perceive this as pain and others as a sensation. If pain is persistent, discontinue use.

Worsened Condition:

If there are any worsened conditions when using the Biomat, discontinue use. Some temporary symptoms may occur, which can be attributed to the detoxification and healing process. For more information, please see the stages of improvement in Richway's Ions and Infrared Rays booklet.

I have added the Foot Chart, that I use, to map the locations of neuropathy in your feet. You can have someone do this for you, so you can chart your progress. Make sure to list the areas that are numb to feather-light touch, and moderately deep touch. It is fun to watch your progress! Get a light blue marker, and color in the areas that are numb. Use another color to make dots where it feels sore to pressure. After you start feeling them change, you can map your progress by going over the blue area with another color, to show where you are now numb. Or, make a few copies, and do a new one for each mapping!

DeLillo / Barefoot Again / 142

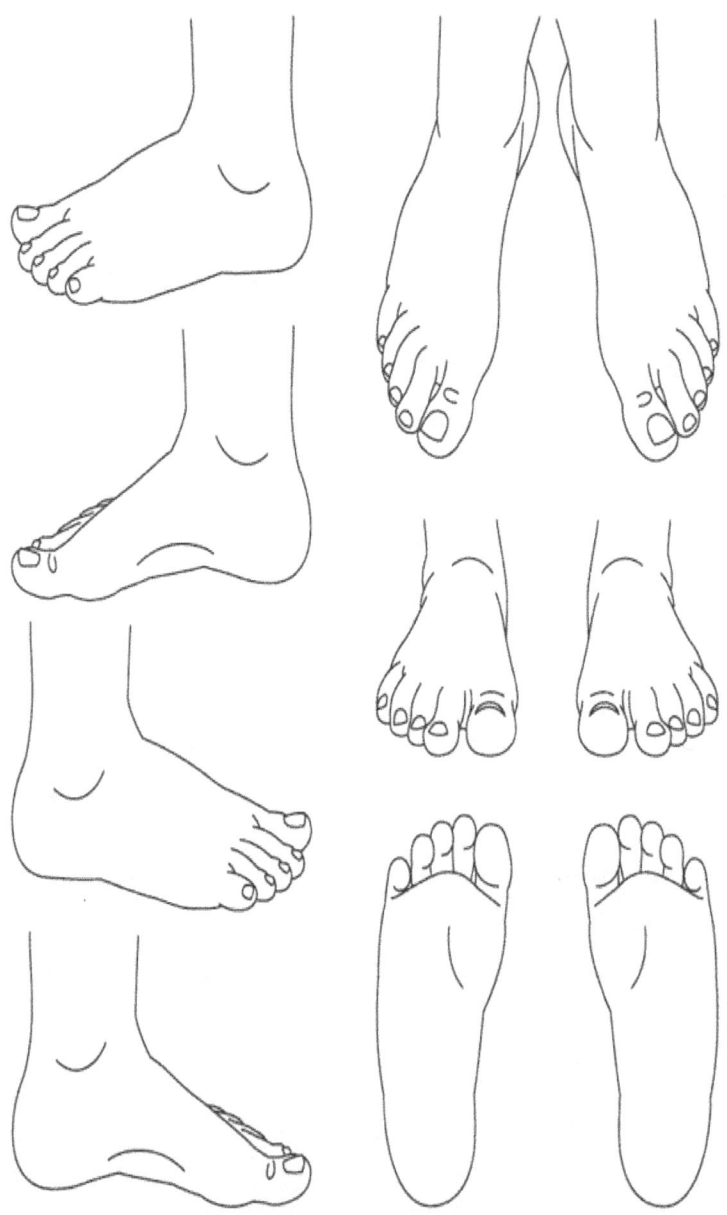

Record Your Journey

Two Week Jump Start	
Sunday	
Monday	
Tuesday	
Wednesday	
Thursday	
Friday	
Monday	
Tuesday	
Wednesday	
Thursday	
Friday	

Notes	
Date	What are you feeling?

About the Author

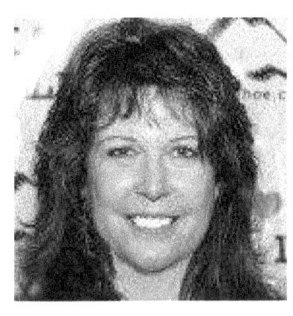

Growing up on the West Coast of America, Mexico and Canada, Roxanne had a rich environment for learning. She was raised by her mother, a Naturopathic Doctor, who spent many years, helping the less fortunate. Even though they did not have much themselves, and often lived in homes without running water or electricity, she found the adventure in every experience. Not that it was fun, just not as bad as some other people had it. One experience that she remembers, and not so fondly, was the winter her mother bought an old Army Officers tent, and pitched in in 6 feet of snow, in Northern Washington. This is where they lived, mom and five kids, all winter. That was a hard year! It did teach all of us about our own inner strength, in adversity.

She started reading from her mother's medical books at the age of four, and would stuff capsules with herbs for her mother. Always inquisitive, she asked many questions of her mom, on why she was using the herbs she chose. If you ask her, she will tell you that she learned a lot from her mom. In truth, she learned a lot of things to do, and not, to do, when it came to health. Her motto is: "Don't over supplement, or go to extremes, just seek balance." She also believes that if you don't know the answer, then don't stop learning, until you do, then, keep up with the newest science, to keep improving.

Roxanne is an Internationally Certified Nutritional Therapist, Master Herbologist, Massage Practitioner, Certified Reiki Master, Animal Reiki Practitioner, Author, Therapeutic Aromatherapist, holds a diploma in Health Sciences, holds Certificates in Lymphatic Massage Therapy, Clinical Foot Therapy, Ebola Awareness and is a licensed OSHA Outreach trainer, Hazmat/Hazwoper Trainer, RigPass Instructor, Medic First Aid Instructor and H2S Instructor. At the time of this writing, she is finishing her doctorate in Holistic Medicine. She is also a student pilot, and wants to someday fly the Alaskan Highway, stopping to camp along the way.

Roxanne has a passion for helping all that come to her, seeking relief. She has been flown across the US, to care for clients after surgery, or that are ill. She has a unique way of caring for people, that instills hope and peace, while going through hard times. When speaking at seminars, she always takes the time to answer all questions. Her wealth of knowledge, on many subjects, is amazing, to say the least.

Little did her first client, with neuropathy, know how profound an impact he would have on her life. From that moment forward, it put her on a journey to either find a cure, or at the very least, a way to improve the symptoms of neuropathy. After a few years of in-depth study, she now has a two week jump start therapy, that helps everyone see improvement in as little as two weeks. Some have complete remission of symptoms, and all make significant improvements. She knew she could not personally help everyone affected by this horrible disease. After many requests, she decided to write this book, in order to give you the tools to help you enjoy walking again.

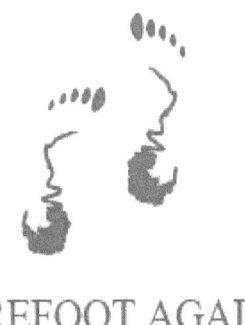

BAREFOOT AGAIN

www.ingramcontent.com/pod-product-compliance
Lightning Source LLC
Chambersburg PA
CBHW050100230526
45470CB00004B/1614